Go ways nobody has ever gone before,

        so that you'll leave traces behind!

For all who escort me on my way...

Regina Lahner

Sound Massage
With Singing Bowls
Easy Done

Theory and Practice

Step by Step Guide

Simply – Clear – Comprehensible

Coverdesign: Friedrich G. M. Roedig, Vallendar

Resources: Own & stock.xchng® vi   www.sxc.hu

Covertext and photo from Regina Lahner: Andreas Marx

Lectorates: Senta Konopke and Anna Lahner

Translator: Dr. Georg Woodman

Bibliographic Information: Deutsche Nationalbibliothek
Original edition: German

ISBN: 978-3-8423-1349-1

1. Edition in English 2016   © 2016 Regina Lahner

Production & publication: BOD Books on Demand, Norderstedt

Important Notice: All made statements in this book are carefully researched and composed; however, author and publisher waive any liability by using directly or indirectly methods and applications of described techniques upon third parties. Whether improvement of personal condition belongs to one's own discretion and responsibility. By any form of health-infringements, especially chronic and/or severe issues, persisting problems, we strongly suggest to seek the advice of a physician (MD) or natural healing practitioner.

About the author: Regina Lahner was born in 1965 in Mönchengladbach/Germany. She's been living since her age of 2 in Bavaria/Germany and occupied herself early on in life with natural healing and all health-related topics. In 2000 she underwent an education-program of 1 year as a Dr. Edward Bach Flower Essence Remedies Therapist, and later on worked independently in the field of advice, education and seminars, and since 2005 she's offered a distant-study program of 10 months to become a Dr. Bach Flower Essence Remedies Therapist. In the same year she accomplished her education „Tibetan Sound-Bowl-Massage" at the Sebastian-Kneipp-School in Bad Wörishofen. As a referent and seminar-chair in the field of Dr. Bach Flower Essence Remedies (speeches/workshops) and singing-bowls (courses, workshops, meditation, and creational sound-painting) Mrs. Lahner is active at numerous public schools in South-Bavaria. For some years now Mrs. Lahner teaches interested persons through intensive-seminars to become Singing-Bowl Sound-Massagists.

Detailed information can be retrieved via www.bluetenberatung.de and www.tibetische-klangschalen-massage.de

Index

Preface	9
Why singing-bowl-massage at all?	11
What happens by a sound-massage?	14
How did singing-bowl-massage happen?	16
The evolution to singing-bowl-therapy	21
Little material-knowledge	22
Treatment and care for the singing-bowls	24
Various sets and shapes of bowls	26
What's needed for a sound-massage?	28
Impact-tools	31
Techniques – Method of striking	34
Ideas, soundplay and introduction	35
Pre-exercises	39
Prepping singing-bowl-massage	41
Please note!	42
Execution of massage	43
Massage in prone-position	45
Massage in supine-position	52

Hand- and Foot-reflex-zone massage	56
Massage w/o physical contacts: Aura-massage	57
Promotion of cognitive senses	61
Play- and exercise-hour with children	63
Fairytales and stories with singing-bowls	67
Meditation with singing-bowls	69
Relaxation and concentration with children	84
Creative relaxation with adults	88
Cognitive sensory perception	91
Cool down after sports	94
Experiences of therapists and applicants	97
Conclusion	100

Preface

I am a quite vivid person, and sometimes, admitted, a rather unrest type. Since that is neither for me nor my direct environment of any benefit I was already early in my life searching for a resting place and a balance. So it once in a while then happened that I took a nap after a stressy day, which led me to meditation or similar relaxation-exercises.

By the end of the 80ies it came to listen to the fascinating sounds of Tibetan singing-bowls which I listened to while I was meditating. (Back in those days just about everything audible was on tape) Well and that then just was it! Even though my tapes later on were distorted through ‚tape-salad' I was retrospectively preoccupied with those sound bowls, and then, short over long, my first set was there!

Sometime later, my two kids were born, and I sought for new goals in my life, and found such after my 1-year-education to become Dr. Edward Bach Flower Remedies Therapist in

2000 I went on to become sound-massagist in 2005.

Since 2008 I've taught hitherto over 300 interested persons from all walks of life the techniques of sound-massage. Besides, at 13 Volkshochschulen (public after-work schools) in South-Bavaria I render courses in singing bowl sound massage.

In the course of time attendees kept asking for literatures. Simple, compact, but able to self-teaching for the private use; but, exactly such book didn't exist as of yet. And that's why I decided writing one.

All these descriptions and observations are based on my very own and subjective judgment, not on any scientific assessments, and ergo don't claim any completeness.

Why singing-bowl-massage at all?

Our audio-sense is of all five, the most accurate.

As daily noise makes us ill, as much it is of necessity to listen to the soft and quite sounds. And that's exactly where the sounds of those bowls help us guide into a sphere of harmony and inner rest.

Each person has over the course of one's life developed one's very own structure of personality; and when in unison with one's environment and in harmony, then, one is content, and, ultimately healthy.

Countless factors (education, school, job, environment...) and the therewith related stress of the day-by-day problems jeopardize our inner harmony and get us off-balance.

In such disharmony we're more susceptible and prone to failure.

- A sound-bowl massage can become your source of energy for the everyday-chores of life.

- Wellbeing, relaxation, wholesome re-creation for body, soul and spirit are quasi guaranteed that way.

The harmonious sounds of the bowls appeal the instinctive trust in a human, they sooth most pleasantly one's dispositioning and the entire nervous system. That way effective relaxation is reached. Each and every of our billions of cells experiences during the sound-bowl massage the gentle swings and reestablishes the original condition.

Self-healing processes can be positively supported that way. During the sound-bowl process deep relaxation occurs resurfacing one's ordered cognitive body awareness, as it takes place in meditation – however here having the advantage that even any layman by hearing consciously the sounds, that way able to quickly turn-off and fall into a relaxed constitution.

In this phase of inner rest lies the problem of releasing problems, tension and blockages (i.e. in shoulder- and neck region) dissolve relatively easy.

Via passive listening and allow-to-happen one enters a meditative state; breathing become deeper, more intensive and relaxed, the muscle-structure loosens, energy-flow "Chi" or "Ki" is being stimulated and existing blockages and tensions can that way slacken, and stress is being combated – which can be observed even after just one sound-massage already.

What happens by a sound-bowl-massage within our body?

When sound-bowls are being placed upon (the usually loosely dressed) body and by means of slightly banging the bowls with a felt-mallet the vibrations of the bowls convey upon the body and spread rippling over the whole tissue.

Just imagine a pebble tossing into the lake – the waves make concentric ripples and widen out over the entire surface, but also below it. And that's exactly how it takes place in/on our body – especially considering that a human body consists to 75%-85% of water, and those liquids, the 'water' enables the vibrations of the sound-bowls to spread out all over.

***Tip:** In case you're already having such bowl you can make that phenomenon easily visible: fill the bowl with water and then dang with the mallet gently the bowl's wall, and the larger the bowl the larger and more intensive are the waves – but careful: it could even spill the water all over!*

Ergo, during such massage the vibrations penetrate deep into the cell-tissue; making one to a body of resonance and part of the sound. It goes without saying that no body is the same, therefore, the sounds vary from person to person, naturally.

And the fact that you'd be seeking for a toilette right after…
If you've had a sound-massage before then you're already aware of the effects. Sometimes midwives use the technique in the effort turning a baby around to give birth to easier.
The effects of a sound-bowl massage ought not to be underestimated therefore!

Attention:
If deemed pregnant do not receive or render any sound-bowl massage! Chronically ill or persons in health-peril, i.e. pace-maker patients, op-screws remaining etc., cancer-patients or any other form of ill-ridden person, they all should consult their physicians prior to any sound-bowl massage consideration.

Now it's becoming historical: how did singing-bowl-massage come to existence and how did happen?

In Asia sound-bowls have been in use in various ways since ages, and the massage with them is an ancient knowledge about sounds and their effects. 5000 years ago already sounds were used in the Ayurveda art of healing in India – and according to their beliefs mankind is made of sound.

Mostly it's Tibet what's considered as the source-country of those singing-bowls. According to legend they originally were used by monks for eating or panhandling, and later on for religious celebrations, where they served the similar purpose as in our regions church bells would do. Later on they spread beyond the borders, where more and more the nowadays sound-bowl massage developed.

About the manufacturing of those bowls one can´t learn a lot. However, the whole procedure is kept secret and treasured.

Small family-enterprises and whole villages and communities produce their bowls based on ancient and traditional recipes.

As well as in Nepal and India those sound-bowls are being manufactured in small factories according to its original Tibetan idol.

They differ from time to time in shape and alloy, however, they're just as qualitative as those from Tibet. Relevant is just one thing: the sound, and the vibration. Age or origin of production, they're secondary – yet later more of that.

What is known is that from an alloy a kind of a flat cake is baked, the cooled – and then the arduous hammering it into a form begins; and up to 30 times the bowl must be reheated, and again via muscle and brachial power shaped, more and more into what's looked for.

Oftentimes even several workers manipulate on just one bowl: while one man turns the bowl by means of using tongs another keeps hammering the walls from the inside with special hammers in a rhythm while sweating heavily. That way the material hardens and dense – and the surface keeps increasing. Another reheating is required to take off the tightness of the material.

Has the final stage –after many hours- finally being achieved, a surface-honing takes place, and afterwards a polishing, bringing the bowl into its final state.

Sometimes bowls are being engraved in an artistic way, or being blackened and cauterized and ornated with symbols, scripts and patterns.
Now the bowls are ready for export into the world.

There are many differences in quality and price. Not always is a pretty bowl also a good bowl. Meaning: the sound and vibration are by far more to consider than looks and price. Some of those bowls are being produced via machines – rendering them oftentimes a pretty look but suffer in sound-quality. Depth of a sound-bowl is produced via hand, not machine.

A layman naturally wouldn't be able recognizing such facts at all, and even more tough since those bowls are being 'treated' by hand afterwards, rendering them the natural and authentic look.

Also, during my research for my book, I've been informed through the grapevine, that some dealers bury their bowls into the soil to affectionate an antique look – duping a customer to have them more valuable and ergo, more expensive, but also better in quality.

Mean. I only can concur such tactics, but can't confirm the better quality at all! Be it now „old", or „young" really doesn't matter; but what does is: sound-quality. But that's not limited to our sound-bowls, is it?

All kinds of musical instruments have better or lesser examples to display; what makes an instrument to a quality-instrument is mainly the manufacturing, use of materials, but not majorly of the year it was manufactured.

And, as many antique vases and bowls are on the market nowadays they couldn't have been produced in ancient days in such number. Since they originally weren't even designed for sound-bowl massage therefore there're just a few original and antique ones remaining, since they'd not even par to today's standards.

Besides that, in the old days a bowl being used for a longer while was usually molten again since it had become unsightly. Since those regions were driven by poverty all material available were used and reused.

The evolution to singing-bowl-therapy

Peter Hess is considered a pioneer in the sound-bowl massage. He's brought the first bowls from his journeys in Asia back to Germany, and already in 1984 he researched the effects of the sounds onto human. He's ergo considered the founder of the after him named massage-therapy: Peter Hess®.

But also other people have occupied themselves with the effects of the sounds onto human beings. Let's therefore name just a few: David Lindner, Frank Plate, Otto-Heinrich Silber, Hans Cousto, Christian Appelt und Jonathan Goldman. Each one of them has experienced their very own approaches und has set relevance into the research of the tones and sounds.

Little material-knowledge

Sound-bowls consist of complex alloys, containing among others:

- Copper
- Pewter
- Iron
- Zink
- Antimon
- Selenium
- Tellur
- Silver
- Gold
- etc....

The already described and arduous production-procedure and the precious base-materials, having silver has the best resonator of sounds, explain ergo the rather high cost of purchase-price.

However, other 'musical instruments' are not cheap either.

Sound-bowls don't undergo any wear-and-tear, and have no further costs, being an investment for life, and can, by care, bequeathed to the grand-children.

All singing-bowls already radiate a certain tranquility just from their outer shape and looks; but once one hears their sound, one feels like in a different dimension.

"So connect our sound-bowls the modern world with the one of Far East and become a unique experience!"

Notice: There could be metals or just traces of those causing an allergic reaction – for that, there should never be stored food in any of these bowls, nor even for re-energizing drinks or so.

IT'S THEREFORE ADVISED TO WASH HANDS THOROUGHLY after any massage and/or protect sensitive people from direct contact to the metals of those bowls.

Treatment and care for the singing-bowls

Such bowl is a particularly special musical instrument, which needs to be treated accordingly.

- Bowls should never be dropped or discharged abruptly

- Since a bowl swings and vibrates it must be placed upon a soft surface, i.e. towel.

- The bowl shall always be danged at softly via felt-mallet.

- A leather-wrapped wooden mallet is suitable for initiating the walls of the bowl, which needs to use a softer pressure outside along the wall of the bowl around. After some exercise you may be able to draw out some swinging/singing sounds from the bowl.

- Never should you use abrasive cleaners; a moist microfabric-cloth with a hint of a detergent is of suffice.

- Larger soiling or some form of oxidation can be solved via „Wiener Kalk", which is a natural cleaner, toxin-free, consisting of ground calcium-magnesium-carbonate and/or kaolin-mill with parts of very fine quartz.

- Pleas dry the bowl thoroughly if they're collected moist on it or you've used it with water.

- For further care you might wish to use a hint of olive-oil to protect the bowls.

- Should it ever be necessary, those bowls might be cleaned through a simple and generic household-cleaner and/or disinfection-spray/cleaner.

Various sets and shapes of bowls:

There are quite a few shapes of those bowls: Indian, Tibetan, Japanese, Chinese, Planet-bowls... those which a driven, poured, engraved, cauterized, glazed, matt, new, antique, and those with higher copper or crystal – who and how would anybody know which one to choose?

My advice: go to a trusted dealer who knows bowls and possibly even the massage-technique. Let him/her explain and demonstrate – and then you make your own selection. Choose what appeals to you intuitively, hit the bowls with the mallet, listen to the sounds, feel the bowls, feel the vibrations, put them onto your body. Take your time to figure out your right bowls.

If you want to select a set for yourself, use a leather-wrapped mallet or hammer and strike the edge of the bowls, and using a wooden hammer the sounds are clearer and harder than with a felt-hammer and the sounds are more precise for the layman.

If nevertheless you'd feel unable to determine you should ask the vendors to put the bowls on lay-away or hold for a few days for you. A good dealer would show understanding.

The more frequent you'll hit the bowls the more intensive are the nuances of sound-variations to you. Listen to your guts-feeling! Of course, not just the sound must be right, the bowls also should appeal to you optically. Don't be misled by the dealer's or other person's suggestions, it must be decided solely by you.

What's needed for a sound-massage?

I'd say, **at least 3 different bowls**
(heart-, joint-, pelvis-bowl) in the middle-weight class. The relaxing sound-flow waving throughout the body cannot be attained with just 1 bowl.

Regardless how many after all, they all must be tuned to each other; nothing could be worse for your sub-conscience waiting for the wrong sound not matching to all the others. Which analogs to an orchestra where one musician plays false tones. Next to tone, vibration and swings ought to match, too.

If you'd like to become more professional on those **a set of 5** (small heart-, large heart-, joint-, small pelvis-, large pelvis-bowl) would be recommendable.

The 3 smallest of all bowls:
(= small and large heart-, one joint-bowl) can be used for a kids-set.

The 3 medium-set bowls
(= small heart-, joint-, small pelvis-bowl) for petit women and youths.

The 3 large bowls
(= large heart-, joint-, large pelvis-bowl) are ideal for tall or/and heavy people.

As a rule-by-thumb guideline using these 3 bowls:

300 – 500 g (heart-bowl)
For the upper body-region

900 – 1100 g (joint- or also universal-bowl) with a broad sound-spectrum for the joints

1500 – 2500 g (pelvis-bowl)
for back and stomach

If initially you'd prefer just 1 bowl, be it financially, I'd suggest taking the universal bowl.

That one can be used "universally": hands, elbows, shoulders, feet, knees, soles, but also everywhere on the body, and for children even as pelvis-bowl.

That one would cost, varying by vendors, ca. 95.00 Euro and up. If one can swing more one should by the entire set of 5; complementing to those are:

500 – 900 g (large heart-bowl)
for the upper body-region

2500 – 3500 g (large pelvis-bowl) with deeper, meditative-relaxing tones.

With the described 5-part set you then can apply massages to kids, youths, light or heavy adults. Size and weights of bowls depend on the constitution of the person being massaged. That makes the massage even more effective, isn't however necessary.

If such 5-piece set bursts your budget you may reduce it to the 3-piece set, which would mean to omit the largest and smallest one from the 5-piece set.

Impact-tools

Each bowl can be influenced by using different hammers. One with felt-cover generates a lighter sound while a larger and softer felt-hammer generates deeper and earthen tones; one leather-wrapped wood-hammer makes the bowls sound cleaner but has less soft volume.

Since now exactly the voluminous tones are the ones desired should for massage-purposes always be used a felt-hammer.

Important: *the wooden hammer is not to be used for sound-massages.*

The deepest sound is generated by the
pelvis-bowl (1500 – 3500 g)
and is being struck with a **large** felt-hammer.

A somewhat higher sound is in the
joint-bowl (900 – 1100 g),
or also called universal-bowl, which would need a **medium-sized** felt-hammer.

And lastly, the
heart-bowl (300 – 900 g)
should have the highest sound and is hit by the **smallest** felt-hammer.

Would you have a small deco-bowl, also called
Zen-bowl (100 – 300 g)
with a bright and clean sound? You can use that one for 'wake-up'-call after the massage, also possible using it during the massage in hover-position of the head to clear one's head.

Note: *Please, never place the bowl unto the head!*

Basic-rules:

The bowls, from small to middle to large, are being hit with felt-mallets also according to small – middle – large.

A practical double-mallet with two different-sized heads (6 cm and 9 cm) is a great compromise and easy to handle, which is best for the sound-massage in my opinion. A complex 3-4 hammer handling is way too complicated. Choose which hammer-head sounds best on which bowls.

Techniques - Method of striking

We understand by that the differing variation in terms of intervals, tact, and strength. Some clients would need a louder and harder and some others again a softer and quieter sound – all depend on one's sensibility, the sound reverberates longer in one's body.

Suggestion: Pay attention to your client's reaction and heed to the individual's needs. I suggest using a silent counting up to 5 or 6 initially until the intervals become automated.

Now try to maintain that rhythm throughout the entire massage. With some more experience later on down the road you'll find the ideal rhythm and don't need to adjust every single time.

***Tip:** If you have a stressed-out or unrest client you should really gently proceed hitting the bowls – and in a drained and exhausted client you could use short(er) intervals in striking the bowls; just listen here to your own intuition.*

Ideas, soundplay and introduction

I've got here some ideas and sound-games for you which you alone, or with a partner, in a group, with kids or the elderly could try out.

Take yourself plenty of time to let the sounds impinge upon all participants.

For that you'd need at least one bowl and several felt-mallets (best in different sizes) and a leather-wrapped hammer or other tools suitable.

> ➤ Experience the properties of the metals first.

> ➤ Aim at the bowl, gently let it sound up. Hold the mallet loosely, strike the bowl at the upper rim softly.

> ➤ Listen to the sound until it fade away.

> ➤ Try and exercise the striking from different angles. How does the tone change? How does it sound best?

➢ How does the tone change when using differing mallets? Use kitchen- or other tools and materials, i.e. plastic, whisker, wood, metal, spoon.

➢ Generate first louder than softer than harder tones.

➢ Fill the bowls with water, rice, sand, strike the bowl, visually experience the vibrations.

➢ Put your hands under the bowl and strike it with the different tools, sense the differences in vibration.

➢ Touch the vibrating bowl with your fingers, nose, and cheek.

➢ Fill the bowl up with water, dip your fingers/hands into the vibrating bowl.

➢ Step into a large bowl while its vibrating; it may be filled with warm water of course.

- Lay or sit on the floor, touch the bowl with the sole of your feet, feel the vibration!

- Massage your hands or feet with the vibrating bowl; this stimulates the reflex-zones.

- Set the bowl carefully onto your belly – feel the vibration reverberating through the body.

- Lastly, put the vibrating bowl near your heart and experience the tingling vibration.

Important suggestion:

- Refrain from a massage when being pregnant!

- Persons with pacemakers should not have a bowl placed onto the body, especially not near the heart. In doubt, please consult your MD.

- Persons with op-screws or –plates, chronically ill or clients with cancer should consult their MD prior to such massage.

- Persons suffering a tinnitus shouldn't receive sounds with inner resonances which could feel unpleasant.

- Never place a sound-bowl on the head! Have it hover above. Neurological processes in one's brain could be affected by the brain's water which would vibrate, and that could cause headache or even migraines.

- Cover the spots of the skin with a cloth where ever a client might suffer from skin-allergies that way the bowls won't come in contact.

Pre-exercises

A partner supine on the floor with closed eyes. Put a bowl onto your own hands and then strike it with a soft felt-hammer from different direction in the room.

Where does the sound come from?

Let the bowls swing out.

Your partner then gives you a sign when the sound has become inaudible.

Approach slowly your partner's body while bowl is swinging; the lead every single bowl from feet to head in close distance over your partner's body (= 10 – 20 cm) back and forth.

In case your partner prefers to sit, no problem, too. Don't remain over the head (it's oftentimes felt unpleasant) – stop at should-level. Then back to the feet. You can surround the shoulder and move rear-side back to the feet.

This exercise serves the own cognitive senses. This 'aura-massage' can be felt if a person is rather sensitive, even without placing the bowls directly.

An extensive description can be found later on page 57.

Prepping singing-bowl-massage

You'd need a warm and quiet room in a pleasant atmosphere, some resting-pillows and a soft surface on the floor.

Should you have problems while kneeling or prefer to receive the sound-massage while standing, a stable table can serve as well.

Ask prior to initiating the massage whether the person prefers to prone or supine.

Also find out if any indication could exclude the application of the massage.

Since a duration of 30 to even 90 minutes might be requested the patient should use first the toilet, and loose attire is recommended; also: no buttons, zippers, jewelries or similar should be worn since it could interfere with the vibrations or cause unpleasant sounds.

To notice – please note!

We apply a relaxation-method serving explicitly the wellness and comfort of the person to be massaged.

We do not treat to heal or improve ill persons – that may only be done by licensed MDs etc. We treat/massage only to improve the general relaxation of the person.

Therefore, during sound-massage there's no conversation and not even background-music, simple for having the client quickly drift into relaxation-state.

However, let your patient know to inform you in case he/she experiences any form of discomfort; that area should then remain off-limit for the singing-bowl massage.

Execution of massage

The now following description should be understood only as suggestions and not being considered too dogmatic.

Important: *This here is for the application of 3 bowls, and should you have just 1 then it's simply required that that one would need to be placed unto the next body-region accordingly.*

Each bowl is being placed and stricken **10times**, within 5-6 seconds interval, starting from the feet up to the direction head.

Later then the direction is reversed. Before setting a new bowl the one used should be gently touched (to illuminate further vibration) so that way not to 'wake up' the resting person.

This step shall be repeated, however, it won't be mentioned again.

The felt-mallet needs to match the bowl-size:

small mallet = small bowl
middle mallet = middle bowl
large mallet = large bowl

If you'd like to deal with several mallets we suggest using a double-sized one; however when using medium-sized bowls another compromise has to be found to test how the middle-bowl sounds best with.

Massage in prone-position

The person to be massaged lies down comfortably on the **stomach**. The hands should possibly rest beside the body.

Begin with the **right sole of the foot**.
The **joint-bowl** is supposed to be placed in that fashion that it covers the largest portion as possible and therefore covering the vast part of the reflex-zones well enough. Heed that you not touching the singing-bowl's edge allowing it to swing freely.

Now the bowl is being struck from middle toward the upper torso.

The vibrations transfer onto the feet's soles and stimulate the reflex-zones that way.
Make sure that swings maintain; you recall the counting-exercise on page 34?

Pay attention that the bowl isn't neither too hard nor too soft brought to swing and remember: "sometimes less is more".

It's sufficient to repeat the striking **10times**, then let it swing out after the last strike.

Now change over to the **left foot** and massage in the same fashion.

After that procedure is also concluded place the bowl on the hollows of the knees and leaves it there for now.

One now kneels or stands next to the patient holding the **pelvis-bowl** in one hand, straightens out the clothes and places the bowl carefully onto the **middle of the back**.

The **pelvis-bowl** now is being struck carefully and gently from bottom to top at the outer edge of the upper third part in a soft rhythm as before already.

After the swings have faded out, the bowl is placed farther up, to the **higher back**.

Now we add also the joint-bowl, which means we strike first the joint-bowl, which is still standing at the hollows of the knees and then we strike the **pelvis-bowl**.
Repeat so 10times.

Tip: *If the joint-bowl seems not to be placed appropriately between the knees you may move the bowl more up, to the thighs, and strike it there alternately with the pelvis-bowl.*

After that place the bowl onto the buttock, at the **coccyx** to balance off the weight on the spine. Both bowls are being struck in alternate fashion.

Now, after straightening out the clothing, the 3rd bowl is being placed **near the thorax** – the **heart-bowl**.

And now all 3 bowls being hit in consistent count-rhythm.

That is meaning, **joint-, pelvis- and heart-bowl** being hit in cycles, gently, gingerly – and make sure that vibration doesn't fades out.

Next replace the **joint-bowl** from the hollow of the knees-region to the **right scapula**; being now that near to the ear, one must strike the bowl extremely gently!

You can hold the bowl in the same manner as it was done at the feet – figure out yourself what's easier.

The same procedure is being done as before in alternation with the **joint-, pelvis- and the heart-bowl**: 10times so.

Now though one ought to follow the flow of the physical meridians, meaning the channels where the acupuncture points are located. That means to strike from the right scapula to the direction of the fingertips.

After vibrations have faded, the **joint-bowl** moves into the **palm** and all 3 are being hit again in same fashion as before.

Please start again with the **pelvis-bowl**, than **heart-** and at last **joint-bowl**.

If the hands are not aligned near to the body, the bowl may be placed onto the upper arm – or the entire step may be omitted.

Tip: *Work in the way of imagining that the vibration from one bowl transfers over to the next.*

After that step has also been done 10times, replace from right palm to the other, the left side of the body. Hereby not stepping over, but walking around the person.

And the same is done from one onto the other shoulder.
Striking the **pelvis-** then the **heart-** and last the **joint-bowl**, beginning from below.

Then, after the shoulder, the **joint-bowl** is placed into the hand-reflex-zones of the **palm** and all 3 bowls sound off again.

After the **joint-bowl** has faded its swings, take it off from the hand and put it aside.

Now, after the entire body from the toes to the fingertips has been vibrated throughout with harmonious sound-waves, we now change the direction of the striking sound.

We start over again, but in opposite order of procedure, namely from the head's direction downward to the toes, striking the bowls again to redirect the generated energy and therefore complete and close the cycle.

Heart- and **pelvis-bowls** remain where they are, but now strike them in inverted direction, from up to down.

If you'd like, place the **joint-bowl** back into its initial position, between the hollow of the knees, while generation a harmonious tri-tone.

After the steps have been done 10times, remove the **heart-bowl** first and then strike only the **pelvis-bowl** – possibly together with the **joint-bowl**.

Then remove the **joint-bowl**, remain only the **pelvis-bowl**.

In conclusion now the **pelvis-bowl** is being placed back into the center of the body and so concluding struck once again.

That way you redirect and guide back the entire energy into the center, and that way conclude the massage in the prone-position.

In case Mr. Patient fell asleep by now, gently wake him/her up and ask to turn over onto the back.

Here now you could conclude the massage completely – and if so, let him/her rest for another few minutes.

Tip: *Never leave any bowl near or onto a patient's body once massage is finished up. The patient, by now perhaps in alpha-phase, might turn and drop the bowls, which that way could sustain damage.*

In case you do decide ending the massage, you can produce a "sound-carpet" – by simply striking all available bowls once more – in greater distance from the patient- for a few minutes, softly, gently......

Let then the bowls ultimately fade out and the patient keeps on dreaming......

But, if you did decide to continue the massage on the supine-position proceed right on.

Massage in supine-position

The person lies comfortably into supine-position, and placing a knee-roll might help, too; as well as a pillow for the neck.

If there's a patient with a swayback an additional pillow will do, perhaps, to pamper your client, pillows under the arms.

We now place the **pelvis-bowl** just about above the **belly-button**, somewhat near the solar-plexus, the gently touch the patient's body and then gong your bowl about **10time** again.

Then move the **pelvis-bowl** a hand-span lower and add the **heart-bowl** near the heart.

Now strike the **pelvis-bowl** below toward head and the **heart-bowl** in same direction, again 10times, gently, softly.

Then place the **joint-bowl** by the **right shoulder** (holding it from the inside with 3 fingers supporting below) and strike the bowl from the bottom upward toward the heart.

Firstly the **pelvis-**, then the **heart-** and lastly the **joint-bowl** alternately in cycles.

Please consider: *"right" is always seen from the patient's perspective!*

Place the **joint-bowl** in the **right palm**, but leave the other two where they are.

Now strike in order: **pelvis-**, **heart-**, and then **joint-bowl** again 10times.

Let sound off the tone of the **joint-bowl** while in the right palm and then switch the sides.

Repeat the same **now left**: put the joint-bowl first onto the left shoulder and then in the left palm, change the rhythm 10times amid the 3 bowls.

After the **joint-bowl's** sound has petered off, place it away.

You may put it below the feet and tune it together with the **pelvis-bowl** once again.

Beware for the changed strike-direction, though!

We have now massaged the entire body from down to up, and no we change the striking direction that way that we start from head toward the feet to redirect the flow of energy and that way complete the circle.

The **heart-bowl** now together with the **pelvis-bowl** from up to down, 10times slightly banged.

Let sound off the **heart-bowl** and remove it then from the body.

In case the **joint-bowl** is still paced between the feet, strike it in alternation with the **pelvis-bowl** and then put it aside as well.

To centralize place the **pelvis-bowl** into the **body's center** and strike it a few times more; and when the sound has petered away place it aside also.

You've got several bowls available?

Then great, build a sound-carpet by using them all, to give your patient the final touch

and have him/her carried away on the sounds reverberating the body.
In time let all bowls sound off.

When you feel the timing is right, and to come to the finale, use the **joint-** or **pelvis-bowl** placed between the feet and strike them hard(er) to earth the person – and then gently let the patient wake up.

Important, though: *In case your patient has to drive home via car, add the session with a bright sound-off, like cymbals, briefly a few times – which serves like a wake-up. Please pay attention to the person's condition before allowing participation in traffic. Ask for the experience made during the session – and that way you can detect whether person "is there" with all senses.*

Hand- and Foot-reflex-zone massage

In the alternative medicine it's know, yet scientifically unproven, that certain points on hands and feet correspondent with our organs and regions of our body; exactly these properties are being utilized when sound-massage is applied.

When feeling fatigued that way the bodily functions can be rejuvenated, and for that experimentally place a bowl unto the palms, or, if supple enough, unto the sole of the feet. Then gently strike the bowl.

For that naturally the **joint-bowl** is the most appropriate one, and the generated sound-vibrations convey onto and into the tissue and skin in a stimulating way.

Tip: *begin at the right side, ergo from the heart away, coming the body to stimulate and adjust slowly to the stimulus; and, if desired, using stronger strikes. However, start gently, though.*

Massage without physical contacts: Aura-massage

Some people are especially sensible or can't agree themselves to a complete sound-massage; and oftentimes elderly are skeptical approaching something new or unknown.

Dementia sufferer or handicapped perhaps might even fear those bowls, can't deal with their sentiments – therefore and in particular, an aura-massage is recommended. But, what actually and exactly is such?

Well, it is known that persons have a field of energy around them = aura, which come from the Greek language and means breath or whiff.

So, we can imagine some kind of halo; however this theory isn't scientifically based or proven, yet. Nevertheless, a vibration is noticeable when bowls are being placed near a person. Therefore, try out, find out.

Procedures:

- Stand a person in front of you.

- Strike softly at the joint-bowl while at the person's feet and move upwards (in the middle of the body) to the knees while remaining 10 cm distant from the person.

- Remain shortly, then move further upward in the middle towards the pelvis, and again remain. When by now the bowl has ceased its vibration strike it again gently.

- Move up to the heart and pause there for a moment.

- In slow move reach to the shoulders, first the right one, then the left – here is where you strike the bowl again, but very softly since we're now near the ears!

- Change to the rear-side and move the bowl horizontally back and forth a few times.

- Move to the neck-spine, then slowly move downward alongside the spine. Remain again in the thorax-region.

- Repeat the same in the pelvis-region of the spine.

- Now proceed centrally down to the knees.

- Conclude the aura-massage in the heel-region.

Notice: *Please do not move the bowl over the person's head! It oftentimes is perceived unpleasant.*

This massage can be done while the person is seated, bed-ridden or ill persons can receive the massage also only on one side, namely the one facing us.

Here proceed in the same fashion:
from the feet toward shoulders, and then, without changing the body-side, run down the same side again back to the feet.

But, please, heed to the person's reactions.

Discontinue instantly when you notice discomfort or even fear in the person.

Attempt anew a few days later…

Promotion of cognitive senses

We are continuously surrounded by sounds of any kind, form and level.
Not few people have problems dealing with the sounds around them, but also to deal with complete silence is strenuous and people can't relax. Also many lost the connection to their own bodies and the alerts it's sending.

By means of singing-bowls and the sound - massage we'd receive the chance regaining our physical cognitional ability.

- In case it's tough for you to relax, turn off any sound-generating devices.

- Try to escape; which won't most likely happen right away. But, there's a way: listen to your breathing, feel the come and go of air in your lungs.

- When you've calmed somewhat place a bowl onto your stomach and let it swing softly.

- Concentrate on what happens to your body, all feelings, emotions, everything.

- Do this little exercise every day; if time is an issue at least then does it before going to sleep.

- Good sleep and inner rest should ensue after a few exercises. After some time that is somewhat programmed in your body and can now be called up for use after having had another stressful day.

Have fun by exercising and experimenting!

Play- and exercise-hour with children

Even little kids are often already unrest, nervous and easily distracted; thanks to an extremely increased media-offer which influences children and don't allow them to rest.

In playful ways of discovering the overtones of the singing-bowls the little ones so can experience an urgently needed and soothing relaxation.

And: Kids just love those sounding bowls, and let them try out the bowls; some hints we've rendered on pages 35-38 already.

More you'll find out now:
Those easy games and exercises are suitable for birthday-parties and even for pedagogic work in kindergartens, elementary-schools or in a sport-club.

Tip: *For therapeutic work with handicapped or dementia-sufferers as well with the elderly can thus be modified for the needs of those.*

- ➤ Begin with a little breathing-exercise so that the kids gain self-awareness.

- ➤ Then the kids should listen into the silence around them. What do they sense?

- ➤ Put one child a bowl into its hand, and let the others place theirs below. Through how many hands can the vibration be felt?

- ➤ Let the kids lie down with their feet forming a circle; stand yourself right in the middle. Strike the bowl. Who feels the vibration? How far does it move up through one's body?

- ➤ Now each kid may put a bowl on their stomachs and hit it themselves. In case there's just 1 bowl, rotate the bowl.

- Read a story while striking the sound-bowl. Let them draw a mandala (circled pattern) or use their fantasy to draw something.

- Should it be unrest play some music and let them dance or frolic to the sound of the bowl's vibration.

- Also, you may sing a song in unison which is in sync to the sound-bowl.

- Tell a short story or meditate while having sound off the bowls. Let the kids keep their eyes shut, that way you direct their attention back to their inner self.

- Depending on age, kids can apply simple sound-massages to each other.

- Especially in the fields of sports sound-bowls are ideal; establish a smaller circuit-training in 2 groups, and after each exercise the bowl must be hit again by the next child; winner is the group who finished the parcour first.

- ➢ By gymnastic exercises or dance you can determine the tact via the sound-bowl. If it's too noisy use a wooden mallet instead.

- ➢ Tossing game: a sound-bowl is placed in somewhat distance to the kids, who now have to toss a small ball into the bowl.

- ➢ Turn the bowl over and allow the children to hit and drum the surface with different things.

- ➢ Hide something underneath the bowl and let the kids guess what it is.

You already can see there are countless ways to imply the sound-bowl and trigger the kids' fantasies.

I wish you a lot of fun!

Fairytales and stories with singing-bowls

Most kids just love fairytales, and almost every tale can be accompanied with a tone from a sound-bowl; even an already known tale could become anew that way for a child.

You could enhance the concentration by placing the sound-bowl right before the kids, and every time a figure of the fairytales is being mentioned, strike the bowl, or, even better, let the child hit it. This as well can be done in groups.

A kind of competition can be set up among those kids by setting a keyword, and as soon as that word is mentioned one strikes the bowl. A building block as a reward is the being awarded, and at the end, the group that accumulated the most bricks wins.

Also, kids can concoct their own tale, or recite one.

That way in young age already the multitasking is being trained, namely in a playful and fun way.

And another possibility: begin a story, but let the kids spin the thread, and after some time, the sound-bowl is being stricken again, and another child continues the story. So you proceed until everyone had the turn telling a story.

You also might want to replace familiar words with tones, and the kids must guess the words.

Example:
„Once upon a time there was a …….. (gong) now fill in an appropriate word, i.e. king, queen, princess, boy ……..

who lived in a ……... (gong) city, kingdom, valley, castle ……..

You see already: thousands of possibilities.

Meditations with singing-bowls

Principally any form of meditation can be used with the singing-bowls. There're quite a bunch of books on the market over "Journeys of Phantasy and Meditations". Let yourself be inspired from those and just copy initially some proper text-line from those books.

Perhaps you might want becoming creative yourself? Why don't you then just write down your very own, proper and personal meditation, composed for your special needs? You'll discover that it can make a lot of fun!

It's logically sensual to utilize several bowls for your meditations. This promotes relaxation and is as well for other listeners much more interesting and divers.

To remember: *If there're no larger number of bowls available you can by means of utilizing different tools generate different sounds of either higher or lower frequencies on just that one bowl.*

Through meditation, especially a singing bowl meditation, we find relatively quickly to the inner center.

Our breathing rate slows significantly, the resting heart rate goes down and we can thus more easily relax and "let go".

Some participants are so deeply relaxed that the content that has been said they afterwards cannot recall, even though they claim to have not slept!

Others doze off even completely and begin to snore...

Preparation of meditation

If you lead a meditation for a group, be sure to come first even to rest!

For this purpose is best suited a ritual with which you are centered, focus, activate their presence and you can arrive in the room.

- Breathe calmly and deeply a couple of times into the stomach and out.

- Take a drop of a quality-enhancing essential fragrance oil (for example, orange, peppermint, lemongrass) and rub it on your hands, the temples or under the nose.

- You may also press even more before the start of meditation a part of the body (for example, the right little finger) gently and activate your subconscious mind as a trigger point set

Explain briefly prior to meditation

- During meditation no talking! (Kids: no playing!)

- During meditation nobody may disturb anyone else.

- During meditation everyone must remain in quiet.

- Prior to meditation one should use the toilet.

Let the participants rest in lying or sitting position! A position needs to be found one can maintain in for a longer while.

Begin with a little breathing-activity steering attention toward one's inner self.

Speak in a sonorous, soft and quiet voice.

Use the personal way addressing one self.

Use just one or two sound-bowls, with deep tones.

What posture/position should be taken?

Your participants should wear light clothing to it, then to make themselves comfortable on a chair or on the floor (on a soft surface, with a pillow and warm socks). A meditation can in summer also be done well while sitting (on a chair or meditation cushion) or lying outdoors.

Whenever it is cooler, however, a blanket is also necessary, though.

The then position taken should not be changed during meditation possible.

The best time for meditation is, by the way, early in the morning, to find serenity for the day, or evening to come gently to rest.

So let's start, participants get comfortable on a couch - or bottom - with a corresponding thereto soft surface to lie down.

This is usually the best option for deep relaxation.

A pillow or a role (can also consist of a towel, jacket, etc. formed) under the thighs, or in addition to the knees relieves the lumbar spine.

If someone tends to fall asleep during meditation, it is often better if one puts on a chair.

Finish and conclusion of meditation

The longer a meditation or sensory journey lasts, the lower often fall participants in a relaxed, trance-like state. Some people even sleep completely. Therefore, it is necessary to end a meditation also so that everyone is afterwards again fully awake and quite aware of himself. This is especially important if your participants have come with a car to you!

I always use to end the fantasy journey a "wake-up formula" (e.g.: I'm going to count to 5) to complete the relaxation phase.

The participant must actively contract his/her muscles and then also freely move around. So he/she has again controlled being led from the relaxation back into everyday life.

Have finally all eyes opened again, I always use a small bowl with a particularly bright sound that I use to "wake up" completing strikes 3-times in quick succession in increasing intensity with a small wooden clapper.

Attention: *This bright tone can easily be received as shrill and unpleasant. Therefore, please apply the small wooden clapper always only to end the mediation!*

You can then repeat your meditation in a few short sentences in your own words again and summarize. So some participants only then realize what they have been unaware of and how deep "off" they really were!

If you'd need more information, I recommend you to steep into my following books, which are available in German and in English:

Regina Lahner
Klangschalenmassage leicht gemacht
ISBN 978-3-8482-0610-0

Regina Lahner
Sound Massage With Singing Bowls Easy Done
ISBN: 978-3-8423-1349-1

Regina Lahner
Meditationen mit Klangschalen leicht gemacht
ISBN 978-3-7322-5500-9

Regina Lahner
Meditation Made Easy With Singing Bowls
ISBN 978-3-8423-4517-1

Regina Lahner
Neue Meditationen mit Klangschalen leicht gemacht
ISBN 978-3-7357-5070-9

Relaxation-exercise

Sit or lie down, most comfortably, then close your eyes.

Breathe deeply in and out, and with every breath you take relax deeper and deeper (strike the sound-bowl here).

Tension your feets, relax them after every exhale (strike the sound-bowl).

Next come the legs – proceed in same fashion.

Now the buttock-muscles.

Following the back-section.
Breathe, exhale and relax. (Strike the sound-bowl).

Next come the abdomens,
and then the arms –
always alongside the sound of the vibrating bowl.

Now clench your hands, exhale, and relax. (Strike the sound-bowl).

The shoulders follow:
shrug, and drop, in rhythm of breathing - and again strike the sound-bowl.

Shape a grimace with your face, relax when you exhale (strike the sound-bowl).

Now your entire body is relaxed.
You must feel great! (Hit the sound-bowl once again).

Tip: *When you strike the sound-bowls for meditation use darker sounds throughout the whole since they're perceived earthier and more relaxing; especially when participants drift off in thoughts those darker tones "bring them back".*

To have change better use different bowls with differing tones, yet however they ought to blend to one and the other harmoniously.

Important: Let the singing-bowls sound off and fade, and don't strike too many bowls at the same time; wait for the next one until the previous ones has just about faded away in sound.

A small example for your meditation suitable for both kids and adults:

Sound-miracle at Dawn

At a beautiful sunny morning you wake up
(dong!)

You're still half drowsy from you dream which guided you through the night.
(dong!)

In thoughts you slip into your shoes which stand right before the bed.
(dong!)

You wrap a cozy blanket around your shoulders and step out into the garden.
(dong!)

Everywhere the thaw is glittering in the sunrays on countless flowers and grasses.
(dong!)

They reflect the world within themselves.
(dong!)

But, what's that?
Didn't you hear something?
(dong!)

Was that perhaps a bell?
(dong!)

Or something else?
(dong!)

Again you hear the beautiful sound……..
(dong!)

Ding, dong, ding, dong……..
(Strike now the bowls several times, softly, gently – let them dim off, strike again)

You now feel cozy and comfy, safe and sound.
(dong!)

You're in the middle of yourself.
(dong!)

You'll indulge on that feeling now for some longer.
(dong!)

And that's where now you use the blanket, spread it, lie on it – take in the fascinating sound.

Ding, dong, ding, dong……..
(Strike the bowls several times)

They sound off again in the same monotonous rhythm.
(Strike the bowls again)

After a short while close your eyes and let your thoughts come and go.
(Strike all the bowls again)

All that burdens you drops off of you, all fears, all worries, all negative.
(dong!)

There's only joy and ease in you!
Ding, dong, ding, dong……..
(Strike bowls now for 1-2 minutes)

With each sound you drift off farther away into a wonderful condition.
(Strike bowls now for 1-2 minutes)

Your body rests heavy and comfortably on the cozy blanket in the soft grass – and you feel safe and sound.
Ding, dong, ding, dong……..
(Strike bowls now for 1-2 minutes)

If there's a question lingering on your mind, ask it yourself now.
 Ding, dong, ding, dong……..
(Strike bowls now for 1-2 minutes)

Now in this relaxed state you may have found the right answer – from your inner self.
(dong!)

Give yourself some minutes.
Ding, dong, ding, dong……..
(Strike bowls now for a few minutes)

You may by now have found your answer, and now focus yourself on the tones again which reenter your conscience.
(Strike multiple times the bowls, but start from dark to light sounds)

You again feel the warmth of the sunrays on your skin, and nearly all dew has dried.
Ding, dong, ding, dong……..
(Strike the bowls, go from dark to light tones…)

It's about the time now for returning to the house, and be ready for a day in happiness, full of energy and new ideas.
Ding, dong, ding, dong……..
(Strike again several bowls, use light sound only)

Dang!
(The light sound bring participants back into reality)

You stretch and yawn……..
and open your eyes.

You look around, and absorb reality again.

Relaxation and concentration with children

Demands on kids, be it in school or even at leger-time, keeps building up. In addition, ambitious parents or grand-parents instead of promoting demanding from the kids:
school followed by homework.

Then: tutoring, theater-play, sports, soccer, ski-gymnastics, tennis-court, music-lessons, pottery...

Oftentimes there's "no time" for anything else.

So that promoting doesn't turn into excess demand you should assure kids having time in suffice for playing, dreaming and relaxing. Kids must digest their experiences in a playful way and need sufficient time for that.

When they learn in young age already to meditate they'll later on in life deal much easier with stress. Relaxation promotes the ability to concentrate much more. It goes both hand in hand.

Ergo, make your kids also mentally strong for their future. Wouldn't you – honestly – not be just as happy about as over a nice picture or a top-place in sports?

It's not necessary having always guided meditation; a simple strike of a bowl can already be relaxing. For that let the child sit/lie on a soft surface/blanket.

Explain the kid it should now pay attention to itself; leave it up to the child where having the bowl placed. Now strike, easy and soft, the bowl.

Tip: *Consider the joint- or a small pelvis-bowl. A too heavy bowl placed on the child might cause great discomfort.*

As a silent exercise you can together with the child take a fantasy-journey through the body.

Start with having the child supine/prone comfortably – and by now place the bowl, then strike it gently, softly.

Ask the child how it feels its body, whether

feeling warmth or cold, how the individual body-parts feel, what the kid can hear, feel, sense or what it's thinking of.

Take plenty of time!

Perhaps the two of you come emotionally closer and lead a dialogue.

Finish that exercise by having the child breathe through more intensely; then let it stretch his/her arms and legs – and render something to drink.

Bigger/elder kids can do the same for writing-exercises, or memorizing vocabulary or formulas.

To distinct, there are 3 kinds:

1. Visual Type

Those kids need to draw or write things down to memorize. The study-material may be written on playing-card sized cards and put into the sound-bowl.

2. Motoric Type

Such kids now need activities for a successful learning process. So, by walking about in the room and striking the bowl one can promote the learning that way.

3. Auditiotive Type

Those kids need to hear everything what's supposed to manifest in the brain, therefore, use a sound-bowl's tone while reading out aloud.

Naturally, there're as well mixed types. Test out what type the kid in front of you is… and let success take place that way.

Creative relaxation with adults

Thinking of relaxation, you most likely think first of massages and meditation, right? That was addressed in this book already.

But sound-bowls offer just way more than that.

You can convert your home-bathtub into a wellness-temple in a jiffy. Each bowl floats on the water, and here can transmit vibrations perfectly. Perhaps even some candle-light?

Let your thoughts go while sounding off the bowls. Yet, do use a rubber hammer or wrapped wooden hammer, if none to your availability, Home Depot etc. can offer such in an array, even though they're going to be misappropriated.

Use an oil or foam in addition to the bath, but no salts. You know what happens to metal and salt: oxidation.

Dry the bowl after the session thoroughly.

To remove any residues from the bowl take some dish-soap.

Having the large pelvis-bowl a foot-bath can serve well and cause miracles, pour warm water and add some etheric oil and a shot milk, cream or whey – which serve as a natural emulsifier. Bathe for about 10 minutes, and strike the bowl from the outside to maintain its vibration.

Proceeding right afterwards to the tub you may add some lavender, Melissa, but if the day is still ahead of you use orange, grapefruit or lemon instead. During cold season or when having a cold you may switch to eucalyptus, teat-tree oil or peppermint.

Pamper your skin with a soothing facemask, so let it take effect while experiencing the vibration of the sound-bowl. Place the bowl right onto your belly, strike it, and the reverberation of swings drift you off…

Do you like the sauna?
Perhaps you or your friends own a sauna? Here too, or in a warming-chamber, those bowls can be utilized and take great effects.
The soft sounds and fine swings promote deep relaxation, and the perspiration-process is being cranked up that way.

Tip: Place all available bowls on a towel onto the sauna-bench.

But, careful! Bowls become very hot!!

Strike the bowls, using a felt-mallet, pour some water over the oven, and fan the hot air.

You may place a bowl into your own -towel-covered- hand, pass by each sauna-user and strike the bowl in front of each one in chest-level.

Pay attention to each one's reaction.

A breathing-exercise or meditation can enhance the experience greatly.

Depend on temperatures in the sauna, don't extend beyond 10 minutes, though.

Cognitive sensory perception in seniors, dementia and handicapped

In professional senior-homes, care-facilities etc. Sound-bowls always find their use. Nonetheless, just as simple can they be utilized in households and private facilities.

And therefore, some suggestions, for individual- as well as group-application:

- Ask a question, i.e., „what belongs in a cake? "

    Strike the bowl for each correct answer (flour, butter, sugar, raisins, chocolate, fruits, etc…)

    And – further questions:
    "What fruits, veggies, colors? ",
    „What names do you know?",
    "What cities?",
    "What countries?"
    etc., etc…

- Playing games like Memory, Picture-lotto, Puzzles or finding words in a

crossword-puzzle, all can be rewarded audibly with a "gong".
Great memory-games and good for cognitive abilities!

- A bowl is struck, and it's being handed over to someone, without interrupting the sound, though.
A game promoting fine-motoric.

- Stand a bowl onto the belly of a patient and place his/her hands right above/beneath and then strike the bowl. The generated vibrations are clearly sensible for that person, but also additionally in the palms since they're near the bowl. An exercise promoting the perceptual promotion.

- A bowl is struck and placed in front of a person, and as long as the bowl vibrates the person may sing some song, or tell a tale, read a book, describe something, spell a word, or so on.
This promotes communicational and speech-expression.

- All close their eyes; let a marble or so roll into the bowl, like in roulette. Let the marble come to rest. When there's total silence everyone may open their eyes again.
  Who can cognize the tone the longest?
  This promotes concentration and differing audibility.

- Let any pleasant music play and hit the bowls according to the rhythm. Your protégé may move around freely, or you assist if so needed.

- Naturally, you may incorporate choreographed moves, dances or movement-games, as well as gymnastics, of course. This promotes motorics and the sense of balance, the equilibrium.

Cool down after sports

Whether you've chopped wood, have run a mile, visited the gym or health-club, or did some gymnastics at home – after any sportive activity especially in health-related sports, or after strenuous activities, harsh use of the muscle-system, gentle & dynamic stretching should occur.

This promotes flexibility and a mobile spine and joints as well as smooth muscle-tissue. Tension is obviated.

There is a difference between active and passive stretching:

By an active stretching (dynamic, soft springing or bobbing) one shouldn't set too intense stretches. First the muscle-corset is being stretched for 15-20 seconds, followed by a brief respite, and repeat the step once again, and again.

By any passive stretching one assumes a certain stretch-position and maintains it for up

to 2 minutes. This can be perfectly escorted with the sound of a bowl.
Strike a bowl in matching time-distances to your stretching-routine.

Also, some meditative music may play quietly in the background.

Do you suffer generally or during and after a workout of (back)-pain? Send your breath by the sound of the sound-bowl right into that hurt area. Via conscious breathing you may send stimulants into that region and cause certain relief.

By the way, even simple gymnastics, stretching, yoga, tai-chi or chi gong etc. can be done with the harmonious sounds of sound-bowls, simply by matching hits of the bowls with the moves of your exercises.

Warning: If you're a beginner and not to astute in exercising, worse, even feeling pain while executing any of the exercises described in this book, please refrain from such and consult an MD for sports or therapist prior who could suggest certain exercises or may be required correcting some of the moves you've executed.

Detailed explanations of exercises would burst the margin of this book, though.

Experiences of therapists and applicants

During the education-period becoming a practitioner I've made contact with various therapists, healing practitioners, medical doctors and other medical personnel from different branches; I received some interesting feed-back that I now would like sharing with you:

A physiotherapist told me he'd be using those sound-bowls by Parkinson-patients; and with astonishment he'd noticed how soon the twitching would cease, as soon as a bowl is placed upon the patient's stomach. The effect was still there on the following day.

Another episode by a successful and versed acupuncturist uses by frightful or resisting patients even before the session some sounds of those sound-bowls already to relax and remove anxiety; with an additional side-effect: the effect of the needles is enhanced through the vibration of the bowls.

A sport-physio therapist, who cares for a soccer- and ice-hockey team and also runs a wellness- and massage-center, told me about a patient who had a burn-out diagnosed, and typical methods were without any avail. The break-through though took place when sound-bowls were used, and that led to a treatment success after all. Convinced over the success those bowls have been used for the sports-teams as well.

Another participant had an operation on her nerve-canals at the elbow. After removing the threads remained a numb and furry feeling. Her treating doctor stated that this could last for 3 or more months. Yet, after just 2 days of sound-bowl treatment she could feel some "zapping" which improved day after day. Her physio-therapist was puzzled and astonished.

The mother of a midget-son shared with me that the daily painful routine of re-adjusting the screws inside her son's leg at the external fixture the bow had embraced the relaxing sound of the bowls being placed onto his belly.

An ergo-therapist explained how one could improve the fine-motoric of a stroke-stricken patient with paralysis when using the sound-bowls.

And, a senior-caretaker told me that they'd be using sound-bowls in their facility for the elderly.

Numerous wellness-massagists, beauticians, chiropodists and pediatricians utilize effectually sound-bowls by having the bowls at the body or feet or even as foot-bath.

Notice: *I'd like to encourage you to experiment a little with these sound-bowls and experience how to maximize effects and areas of use – and record your experiences.*

I'm looking forward to receiving your reports!

Conclusion

Such sound-bowl is not just a decorative thing, it can, as you by now know, be quite versatile.
Outstanding in its use for meditation, partner-massage or even self-massage.

In nowadays' hectic time we live it becomes more and more important to relax; some even take their jobs home or into their leisure, rush through the landscape with a timer, and now think they'd be doing themselves a favor and relax.

What you and especially your body really needs is genuine relaxation, to switch off. As a stressed person one needs to learn again to focus on one's inner self, to recognize the orchestra of function among body, spirit and soul; and, to accept such.

Already 1 ½ centuries ago, the 'water-doctor, „Wasserdoktor", Pfarrer Sebastian Kneipp (1821-1897), used to say:

„*Who doesn't invest time for one's health must one day sacrifice a lot of time for the illness.*"

(Wer nicht jeden Tag etwas Zeit für seine Gesundheit aufbringt, muss eines Tages sehr viel Zeit für die Krankheit opfern)

Many therapists (i.e. physiotherapists, ergotherapists, speech-pathologists, healing-practitioners, and even MDs) meanwhile have been committing themselves in their daily work by using sound-bowls specifically.

The patients profit from the relaxing effects of the sound-bowl massage, the tones attract the subconscious, promote inner recognition and the vibrations can even promote the powers of self-healing.

In the field of care from kindergarten to schools up to senior-centers, at work with the ill, handicapped, and dementia-sufferers sound-massages and games with singing bowls can be very well incorporated into daily activities.

All mentioned application-possibilities and – options are based on long-years experiences made by those who have used the sound-bowl massages.

Nonetheless, different reactions and individual effects are possible, since every person is indeed different and ergo reacts differently upon the sounds and vibrations of those bowls.

When you may have enjoyed my book I'd be more than happy seeing you in one of the sound-bowl massage intensive-courses, meet you in my distant-learning courses to a Dr. Edward Bach Flower Essence Remedies Therapist, or in any of the other courses and seminars I offer and hold in Germany.

All current dates you may find on the Internet at the German pages
www.tibetische-klangschalen-massage.de
and
www.bluetenberatung.de

Have lots of fun in experiencing your own sound-bowl massage!

That wishes you

Regina Lahner

Do you own a Smartphone?

Using this QR-Code you can call up further information: (in German language)

Homepage
Singing-Bowls

Homepage
Dr. Edward Bach Flower Essence Remedies

Twitter
News